BALD IS BEAUTIFUL

BALD IS BEAUTIFUL

WILLIAM P. TAYLOR

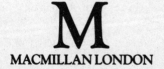

MACMILLAN LONDON

First published 1983 by

MACMILLAN LONDON LIMITED
London and Basingstoke

Associated companies in Auckland, Dallas,
Delhi, Dublin, Hong Kong, Johannesburg,
Lagos, Manzini, Melbourne, Nairobi,
New York, Singapore, Tokyo, Washington
and Zaria.

Reprinted 1983

Printed in Great Britain by
The Anchor Press, Tiptree

Picture Acknowledgements

Associated Press (USA): 75 right. Canapress Photo Service (USA): 20
22, 24 below, 30, 47, 66, 68, 73 left, 76, 85, 88, 92. Camera Press: 15, 63.
Frank Dickens: 43. Mary Evans Picture Library: 48, 51, 86. The
Kobal Collection: 69, 82. The National Gallery, London: 81.
New Yorker Magazine, Inc: 10 drawing by Nankoff © 1979, 17 drawing
by Ho Martin © 1979, 40 drawing by Lorenz © 1974, 54 drawing by
Ross © 1976. Popperfoto: 8, 12, 24 above, 25, 26, 27, 33, 41, 55, 65, 71, 72,
74. Rex Features: 31, 36. Dan Sherbo: 79. Sporting Pictures (UK):
60, 62, 64, 75 left. © 1982. United Feature Syndicate Inc: 73 right.
Universal Pictorial Press and Agency: 38. Van Nostrand-Rinehold: 34.
© Laurence Whistler 1946 and 1978/John Murray (Publishers) Ltd: 87.

Jacket Illustrations by Frank Dickens.

'It is ironic
that a man should consider
his bald head a sign
of lost virility,
because it is precisely
a man's maleness
that helps to make him bald.'

SYLVIA ROSENTHAL in *Cosmetic Surgery: A Consumer's Guide.*

Contents

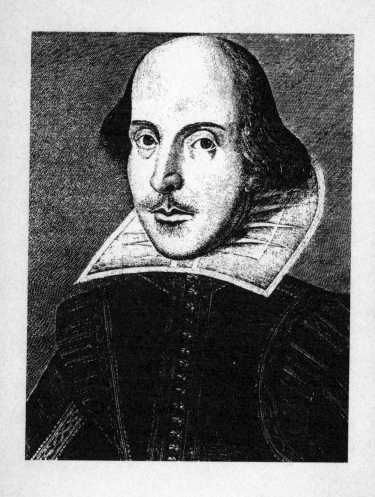

What He hath scanted men in hair,
He hath given them in wit.
WILLIAM SHAKESPEARE

DEDICATION
Hair! Hair!

Hats off to the hundreds of thousands of handsome, virile, and – let's face it – just plain sexy men who are born without hair or who, since birth, have lost enough of it to be considered bald.

Yes, bald!

Not balding, or thinning, or receding, or sparse . . . but bald!

Beautifully Bald!

This book is written for, and dedicated to, you.

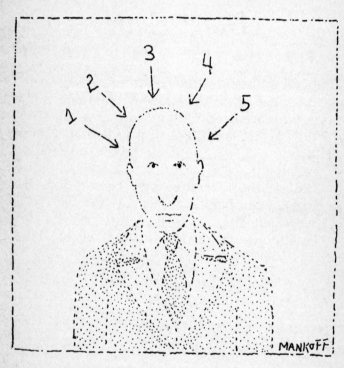

The Five Major Warning Signs of Baldness

The Bare Facts

It is entirely possible to keep your hair from falling out by taking oestrogen shots (female hormones) to balance the testosterone coursing through your body. The therapy, however, does have its drawbacks. For starters, your voice will change. And then in fairly rapid succession, your dink will shrink, you will undoubtedly develop a beautiful complexion, and finally, you will grow breasts.

Testosterone, you see, is the male hormone. The one you probably *least* want to 'balance'. It's the one that gives your voice that John Wayne edge of authority. (And he was bald!) It's the hormone responsible for the fact that you have to shave every morning. It makes your chest and pubic hair grow and probably goes a long way towards explaining why you prefer martinis, whisky or beer to white wine spritzers or crème de menthe frappée.

In the foetus, testosterone is responsible for the development of external genitalia, and later, at puberty, for the continued growth of that equipment.

In short, it determines the cut of your jib – it's the thing that makes a man of you.

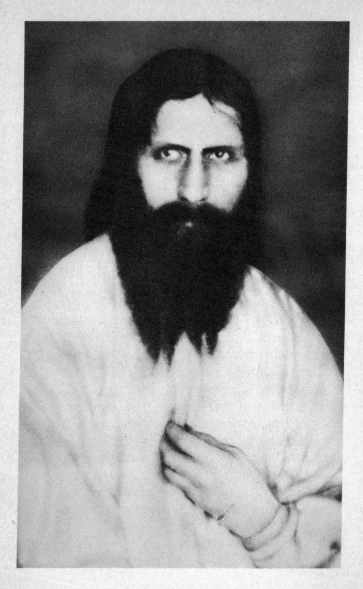

And it is precisely a man's maleness, according to leading dermatologists around the world, that helps to make him bald.

To promote this fact, and to lay to rest the various hair-brained and fuzzy-headed theories about baldness that have sprung up over the past several thousand years, is precisely the purpose of this book.

Ten things, for instance, which do not cause baldness, are:

- Homosexuality
- Banging your little noggin against the head of your crib as a child (Rasputin did this and was frequently mistaken for an animal)
- Banging your brains out against the head of your bed during sex
- Masturbation (it's a well-known fact that masturbation grows hair, albeit on the palms of your hands)
- A low IQ
- Wearing too-tight jockey shorts
- Not wearing a hat in winter
- Premature ejaculation (King Kong couldn't even *look* at Fay Wray without practically drowning innocent bystanders, and never lost a hair in his life)
- Watching *Match of the Day*
- Booze

On the other hand, ten things which undoubt-edly assist your testosterone in speeding you along the way to manhood – ten things, in fact, which probably mean you are getting there much more quickly than you ever dreamed possible – are as follows:

- Heredity (beautiful parents are much more than the luck of the draw)
- A keen wit and sense of humour
- An inquiring mind
- A large penis for your age, weight and height
- An almost fanatical desire to have women experience orgasm before you do
- A remarkable and outgoing personality
- The ability to solve problems easily
- Success
- You seem to have more money than you know what to do with
- A sexy voice

So read on.

In the following pages you will find answers to questions you never thought to ask.

Why no one ever heard of Picasso, God, or Yul Brynner until they were bald.

Why Moses was able to part seas, while others sat about parting their hair.

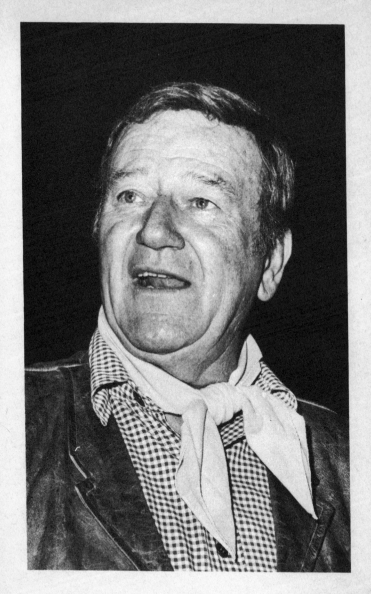

The origin of expressions such as 'Off the top of my head', 'Waiter, there's a hair in my soup', and 'Bald is beautiful'.

We will examine the Samson myth – a bald-faced lie if ever there was one.

We will explore the latest theories about MPB (Male Pattern Baldness) and ISD^2 (Increased Sexual Drive/Desire).

And we will learn why Telly Savalas and Mohicans shave their heads. Why Cleopatra, Daddy Warbucks and the American Bald Eagle preferred to look the way they did.

. In this book, the hair-raising facts about the world-wide conspiracy that has kept the bald and the beautiful out of the romantic-lead and hero roles in *Mills & Boon* novels, movies, television, and even horoscopes. (What's so special about a tall, dark stranger?)

We will examine the all-too-obvious token-ism apparent in such productions as *Kojak* and *The King and I*.

We'll look at Socrates who thought (or knew?) that hair-loss is caused by too much sex.

We'll look at *cures*, and million-year-old recipes.

We'll look at beards.

We'll look at Duncan Goodhew – in the water – and Bobby Charlton on dry land.

Masters with Johnson.

Toscanini with his baton.

Zero Mostel.

Let's look at Roy Jenkins and the SDP.

The hairstyle of Robert Robinson.
What about Clement Freud?
What about Henry Miller?
What about Grace Jones?
And finally, like that nice little bald guy in the trench coat at the edge of the stage, let's yell *'Take it off!'* to every Tom, Dick, and Hairy in the world.

In the words of *The Bald Headed Men of America*, 'If you haven't got it, flaunt it!'

Or, as Janis Joplin sang it better than anyone else, 'Freedom's just another word for nothin' left to lose.'

Go for it!

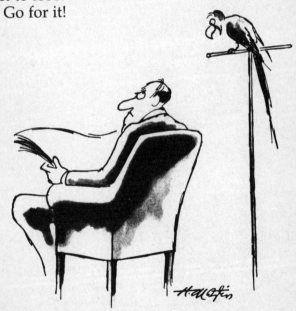

"How about a cracker, Baldy?"

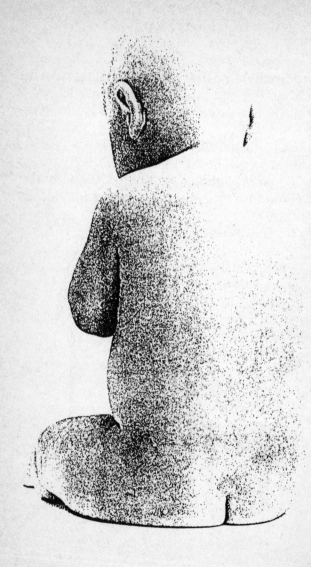

1
We All Start Out Beautiful

In an exchange with Lloyd George at the time of Diana Churchill's birth in 1909, the proud father, Winston Churchill, boasted that she was 'the prettiest child ever seen'.

'I suppose, then, she looks like her mother?' Lloyd George replied.

'No,' said Winston, 'she's the image of me.'

Another story, perhaps the same one altered through retelling, has Churchill, then Prime Minister, approached by a jubilant Londoner as he was leaving No. 10 Downing Street.

'Oh, Mr Prime Minister,' the lady beamed, 'my daughter has just had a bouncing baby boy, and he looks exactly like you!'

'Madam,' he said, pausing only briefly to acknowledge her joy, 'all newborn babies look like me.'

'Baldness,' says television's Kojak, Telly Savalas, 'takes us back to Day One and the way we looked when we first came into this world. "Bald is Beautiful" was the first comment we made.'

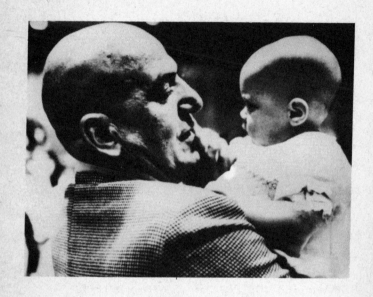

2
Heads of State and Other Beautiful People

Throughout history they seem to rise head and shoulders above their contemporaries.

On the world-stage of politics it is difficult not to compare the dynamic and balding Julius Caesar to that hirsute horde of assassins who did him in.

The bulldog baldness and determination of Winston Spencer Churchill will forever stand in contrast to the hairy and evil madness of Adolf Hitler.

America, when it slows down enough to think about such things, must always mourn the dignified and moral conscience once a hair's breadth from its fingertips in the person of Adlai Stevenson.

Even the Kremlin seems somehow less approachable minus the chrome-domed and gramps-like Russian caricature of Nikita Khrushchev.

And then there was Ike.

We must be careful not to go overboard, to find ourselves promoting theories of bald

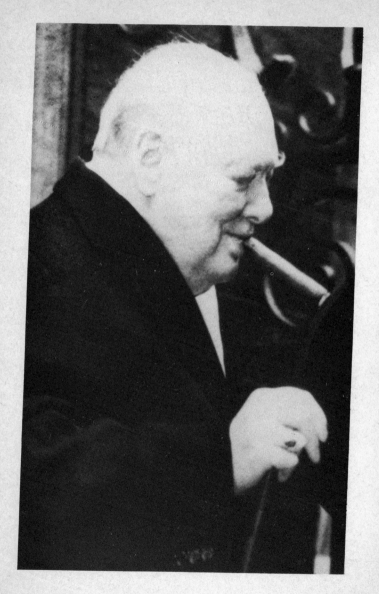

supremacy, but it is hardly splitting hairs to note the disproportionately large representation of the bald and balding among the leaders, generals, statesmen and thinkers of history, and of our own time.

Consider, if you will, the following:

King Solomon
Ed Koch
Mahatma Gandhi
Gerald Ford
Benjamin Franklin
Tutankhamun
Elizabeth I
Vladimir I. Lenin
René Lévesque
John Glenn
The Dalai Lama
Menachem Begin
Edward VII
Moses
Haile Selassie
Charles the Bald
(grandson of Charlemagne)
Chiang Kai-Shek
Henry Adams

Quite a collection, I think you'll agree!

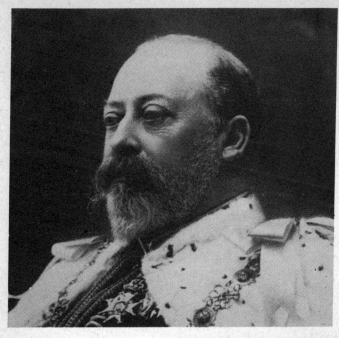

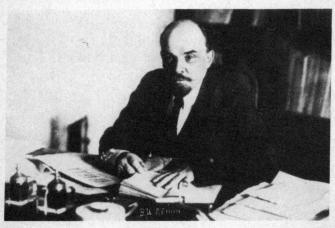

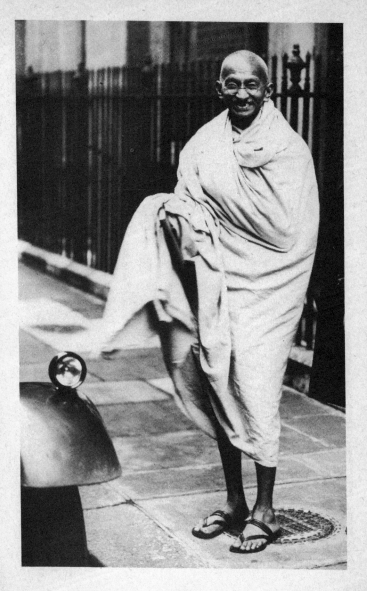

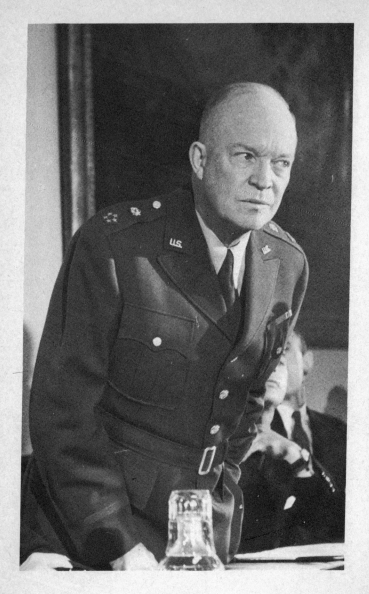

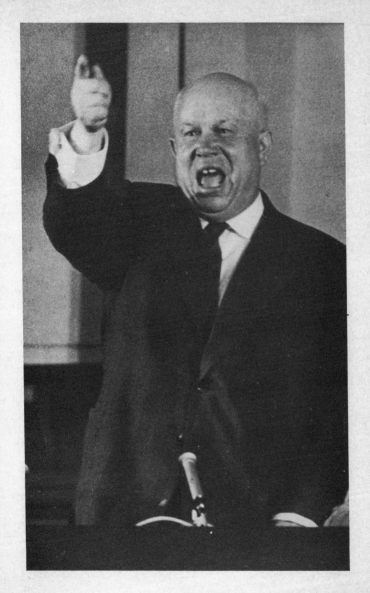

In the worlds of music, literature, the performing arts and business too, still others emerge as shining examples of people at the top of their form.

One need not ask, for instance, what the following have in common above and beyond their well-known faces.

William Shakespeare
W.C. Fields
Aristotle
Auberon Waugh
Pablo Picasso
Louis Armstrong
Socrates
Otto Preminger
Pablo Casals
J.P. Morgan
Daddy Warbucks
Frank Sinatra
William Wordsworth
Zero Mostel
Clement Freud
Toscanini
Bing Crosby
Alfred Hitchcock
William Randolph Hearst
P.G. Wodehouse
Isaac Hayes
Robert Morley
Ed Asner
Hippocrates

Count Basie
Malcolm Muggeridge
John Wayne
Salman Rushdie
Rockwell Kent
Sean Connery
Thomas Keneally
Burl Ives
Allen Ginsberg
Clive James
Elton John
E.T.

The list goes on.

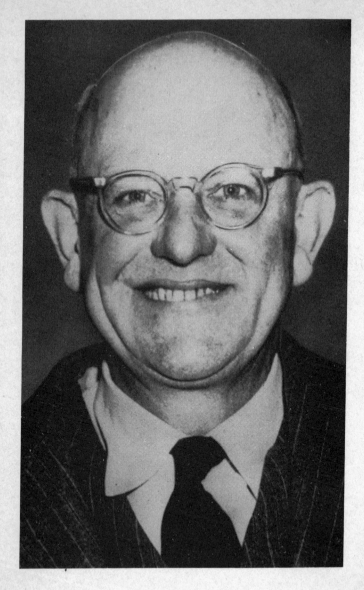

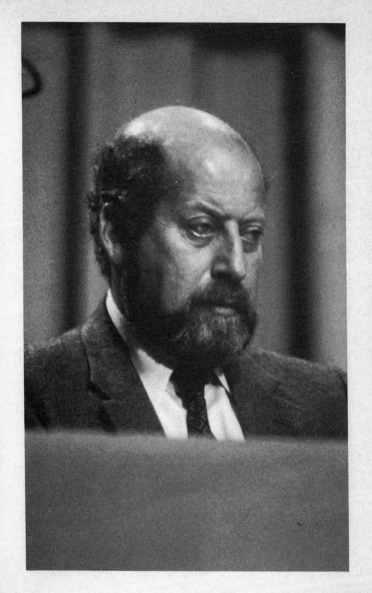

His heed was ballid,
that shoon as eny glas.
CHAUCER

3
Bald as a Genius

The origin of common expressions is a fascinating feature of any language. So too is the consistency with which certain words are used to illustrate certain attributes or features. *Bright as a button* and *Let me unbutton your fly*, for instance, as opposed to *Dull as dishwater*, or *Waiter, this soup tastes like dishwater*. Fascinating, then, to look at the wealth of expressions which have sprouted round our shiny heads, as opposed to those which have taken root around the fuzzier variety. Let's take a look.

Heads I Win!
Good Head
Heads of State
Head of His Class
Head and Shoulders Above All the Others
Head Start
I Can't Get Her Out of My Head
Heads Up
Head Boy
Head Girl

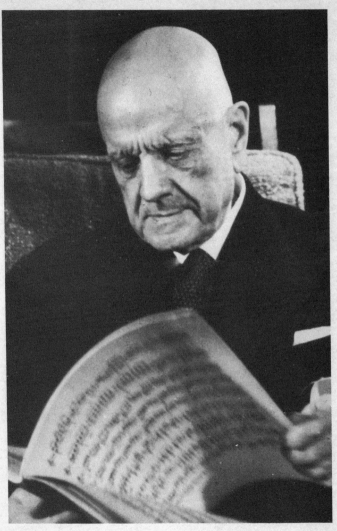

Sibelius – a composer of great genius,
and very little hair!

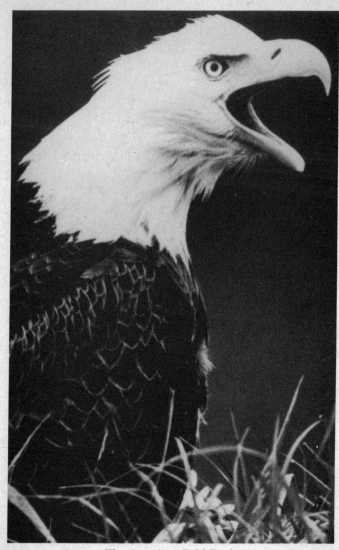

The American Bald Eagle

Corporate Head Hunters
Head of Government
Getting Ahead
Miles Ahead
Who's Going to Head Up That Project?
Let's Head for Town
Head 'em Off at the Pass
Who Heads Up Your Organization Anyway?
That Guy's Got a Head on His Shoulders
Who's Ahead?
Head Over Heels in Love

As opposed to:

Hairy
Hairy as an Ape
Head Full of Hair (as opposed to ideas, we
presume)
Long-haired Hippy Freak
Hair-brained Idea (often misspelled)
Dull as Hair
Waiter, this Soup Tastes Like Hair

But enough. We've made our point. Why,
even if you have just begun to lose your hair,
and people refer to it as 'thin' – think how much
better off you are than having people think of
you as 'thick'.

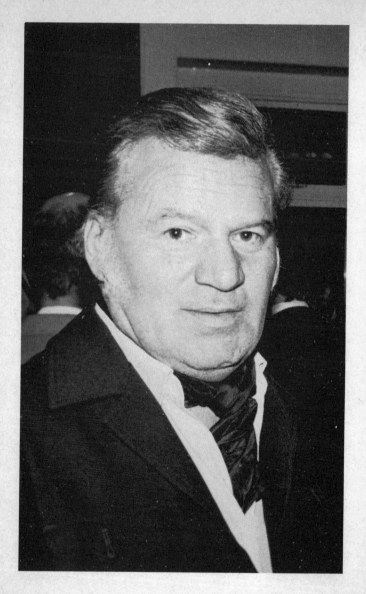

> *Drunk*:   Shay . . . the top of your head
>   feels like my wife's breast.
> *Gentleman*:   By God, it does!

4
On a Wig and a Prayer

To be bald, beautiful and sexy at the same time
is not as easy as it looks. For starters, there are
hairy-assed merchants out there, and harried
advertising executives – a multi-million-pound
lobby that would have us all walking about, our
heads buried under millions of dead hair cells,
our medicine cabinets bursting with embalm-
ing creams and other cosmetic bric-à-brac to
keep our hair looking 'wondrously alive'.

Then there's the basic problem of leaving the
flock. You've been a sort of sheep until now –
your maleness and your individuality safely
hidden in the hair-style of the day – and you
begin to stand out in the crowd. Suddenly, in
short, you are *the man*.

And finally, there are all of those interesting-
ly more aggressive, more demanding, more
fascinating, experienced and slightly frighten-
ing, older women.

No small wonder then that the ranks of the
bald and the beautiful have been thinned of the
following types.

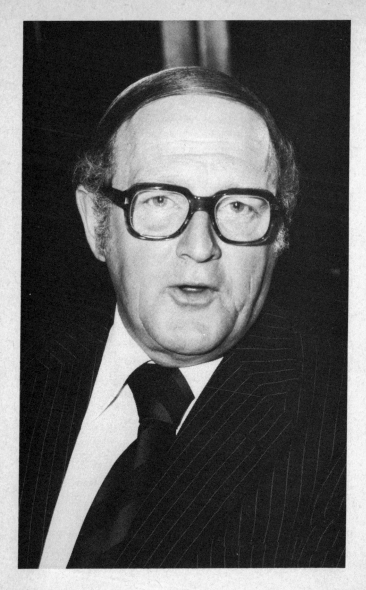

The Sidewinders: those pitiful buggers who would rather drag one, two, or three lonesome strands of hair back and forth, and around and around their heads, than admit to their maleness.

The Wig and a Prayer Set: 'One Colour – One Size – Fits All!' – those poor devils in those shaggy, reddish-brown rugs who would rather spend £99 on a wig than bare anything close to £100 worth of sex appeal.

Touché! Toupee!: and here the rug merchants really clean up! Here's that life-like sod from the other side of the fence – some part of an acre of dead hair cells from God knows where – or what – or who!

This is the £10,000 wig – usually found atop the £10 personality.

Rug Around the Clock: The inventors of 'a rug for all reasons'. Undoubtedly the crowd that simply got tired of saying, 'I just washed my hair, and can't do a thing without it.'

Now they have it!

Happily Harried for the office.

Afro Disco for a night on the town.

Oh, what a Night that Was! (A carefully tousled look for the morning after)

Greasy Gaucho.

Randy Ringlets.

Very Vaseline.

Wet Look (for the beach) . . . *Dry Look* (for after a shower).

These guys got it!

And how!

The Mad Hatters: Jimmy Durante was seldom seen without one. Sam Snead's became his trademark, both on and off the fairway . . . Tom Mix, both on and off his horse. Roy Rogers too. Sinatra, Crosby and Elton John before they swapped for cover of another kind.

And Yasser Arafat and Santa Claus!

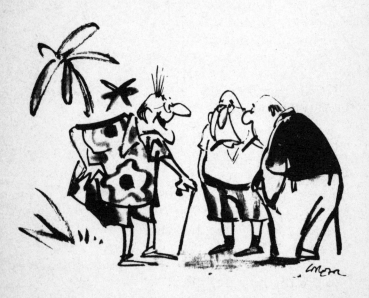

"Isn't it fantastic? They take these plugs from the back of your neck and put them on top of your head, and six months later it's a whole new ballgame."

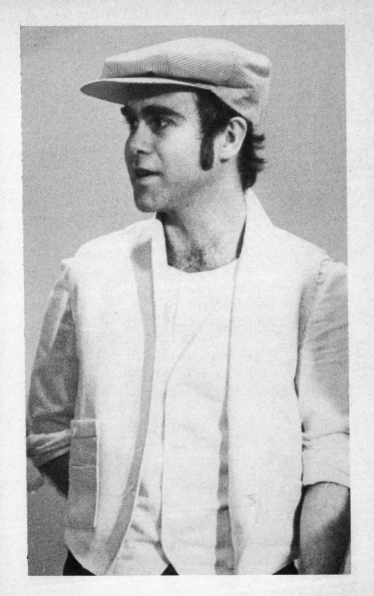

The Conservationists: these are the guys you really worry about. You see them in restaurant washrooms. You imagine them in front of their mirrors every morning – nostalgically brushing and combing . . . and combing and brushing . . . and combing and combing what looks, at best, like some tiny island of armpit that has mysteriously made its way on to the tops of their heads.

Which brings us logically and finally, of course, to the *Cede and Reseed Crowd*. Men so intent on hiding their maleness that they submit to transplant surgery – spending £10,000, £15,000, and even more on their very own, one-man reaforestation projects.

The brochures make it sound simple enough. 'Small, round tufts of hair-bearing skin are removed from the sides and back of a bald person's head. Then, like tiny potted plants, these little clumps are transferred to new little holes punched out in the top bald area.'

What they don't tell you is enough to drive you mad.

Does it need watering?

Does it need manure?

Do you have to dust it against the dreaded boll weevil?

5
And Quiche
Won't Grow Curls

Women have long hair.
Men have short hair.
Real men have no hair at all.

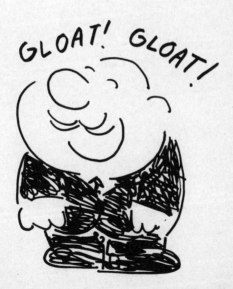

6
The Ten Worst Bald Jokes in the World

Hey Baldy!
Hey Curly!
Hey Chrome Dome!
Hey Skin Head!
Hey Billiard Ball!
Hey Bowling Ball!
Hey Egg Head!
Hey Shiny Top!
Hey Hairy!
Hey Kojak!

7
The Best Bald Joke in the World

A young man enjoying, but not yet totally comfortable with his baldness, is being constantly hassled and put upon by the 'entertainers' at the nightclubs he enjoys frequenting with his many women friends.

Everywhere he goes, the M.C., the stand-up comic or the drunk at the next table rolls out a pathetic liturgy of one-liners.

'I'd now like to do a song for the lady with the curly-headed gentleman at table seven.'

'Well, I see we have a good crowd with us tonight . . . and I'd especially like to welcome Mr and Mrs Kojak!'

'Why did the chicken cross the road? And speaking of eggs . . . do you see what I see at table six?'

Finally, able to take it no longer, the young man bundles up his belongings, takes his hard-earned life-savings, and spends the entire bundle working with the best gag writers in the world.

He studies with top writers, apprentices with the people who wrote stuff for Jack Benny, Bob Hope, and the Two Ronnies. He works out with Dave Allen, George Burns, Morecambe and Wise, Spike Milligan, Les Dawson, Paul Hogan – the lot!

And finally, he returns home . . . most of his small fortune spent, but filled to the brim with new-found confidence.

That very evening he picks up his favourite lady friend, and heads for his favourite night-spot for dinner and dancing.

And wouldn't you know it!

The house lights dim, the orchestra strikes up a familiar tune, the M.C. runs out on to the stage, and, in his very first breath, calls out to the stage manager: 'Arnie, could you please dim the lights just a little bit more? . . . I seem to be getting some reflection or glare from this table down front.'

The usual round of laughter, of course, but even before the M.C. can muster his customary 'Thank you Arnie, that's better', our friend is on his feet – and, with a sly wink at his date, he takes a deep breath and hollers 'FUCK OFF!' at the top of his voice.

Now *that's* funny.

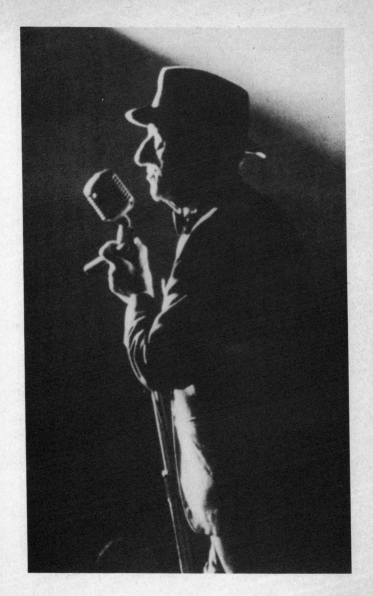

I WAS BALD.

I was born in 1852, and, just as my photograph shows, I now have a full growth of hair. Yet thirty years ago I found scurf upon my scalp, and my hair began to fall away, until after a while I was classed as a "bald head."

Call it vanity if you will, it was displeasing to me to remain bald. Furthermore, I believe it is our birthright to have plenty of hair upon our heads.

Seeking a Hair Growth

It is scarcely necessary for me to state that, in the hope of growing new hair, I had experimented with one thing and another—the usual array of lotions, pomades, shampoos, etc.— without getting any benefit. At that age I looked older than I do now. Later, when I became a trader in the Indian Territory of U.S.A., some of the Cherokees jocosely called me "the white brother without a scalp lock."

American Indians Never Bald

I never saw a bald Cherokee Indian. Both braves and squaws almost invariably use

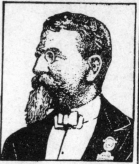

(From a recent photograph)

tobacco, eat irregularly, frequently wear tight bands round their heads, and do other things which are commonly ascribed as causes of baldness. Yet they all possess beautiful hair. What, then, is their secret? Being on the spot—most of the time at Tahlequah—and upon very friendly terms, it was easy for me to gain information from the usually taciturn Cherokees. I learned exactly how American Indians grow long, luxuriant hair, avoiding baldness and eliminating scurf or dandruff.

My Hair Grew Again

Then I applied these secrets to myself, and my hair began to grow. There was no messing or trouble about it. The new hairs emanated from my scalp as profusely as grass grows on a properly kept lawn. I have had a plenitude of hair ever since.

Numerous friends of mine in Philadelphia and elsewhere asked me what had performed such a miracle, and I gave them the Indian elixir. Their hair soon grew over bald spots. Scurf disappeared wherever it existed—

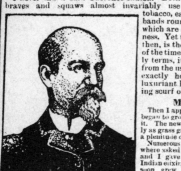

(From a photo when bald)

and it never returned. That these persons were amazed and delighted is stating the fact mildly. The hair that grows is strong and silk-like. It has beautiful lustre, and imparts the appearance of health and vigour.

Do You Wish Hair Growth?

Having established London headquarters, I now give notice that you may obtain Ko-tal-ko at any good chemist's or drug store. After buying it, apply regularly, and watch the result. You are likely to be astonished and delighted, particularly if you have tried various liquids, lotions, etc., without benefit. Or, if you would like a testing box by post, send sixpence (P.O. or stamps of any country) and you will receive the box, descriptive pamphlet, etc., post free.

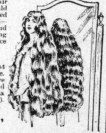

Address: JOHN HART BRITTAIN, Ltd., 2, Percy Street (54BL), London, W.1.

> There is more felicity
> on the far side of baldness
> than young men can
> possibly imagine.
> LOGAN PEARSALL SMITH

8
There's the Rub

Of all the remedies, treatments, and purported cures for baldness which have kept entire populations scratching their heads throughout the history of man, none in recent memory comes close to topping the topping recommended in the Ebers Papyrus dated 1550 BC.

> Apply a poultice of equal parts
> of the fats from the ibex, lion,
> crocodile, serpent, goose and
> hippopotamus . . . together with
> the burned prickles of a hedgehog
> immersed in oil, fingernail
> scrapings and a mix of honey,
> alabaster, and red ochre.

'All with proper incantations', it concludes.
But of course!
Pale, indeed, by comparison, those relatively contemporary lanolin advertisements which appeared in men's magazines under the head-

line 'Have You Ever Seen A Bald-headed Sheep?'

And while Socrates and Hippocrates may have disagreed – the former boasting baldness as the result of too much sex, the latter promoting a 'cure' composed of horseradish cream and pigeon excrement – one fact remains. With 100 per cent of men (and a surprising 85 per cent of women) losing their hair as they grow older, sexier, and more mature, there is a certain inevitability about the fact that there always was and always will be a goodly number of hairy hustlers ready to treat the condition as nothing more – and nothing less – than a cash crop.

Where did it start?

One twelfth-century remedy in the School of Salerno's medical dictionary, published sometime between 1095 and 1224, states: 'For ointment – juice of onyons is assigned to heads whose haire falls faster than it grows.'

More recently, the Upjohn Corporation of New Haven, Connecticut, hired a skin specialist and nineteen doctors to look into the fact that patients taking the drug Minoxidil, for high blood pressure, had began to sprout hair.

In Caesar's day, the Romans swore that berries of myrrh, rubbed into a bald or balding pate, would see it sprouting a lock or two.

And daily since, every age has brought forth potions, ointments, poultices and creams, all aimed at the business of restoring hair or

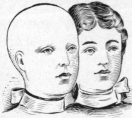
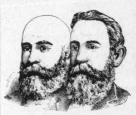
preventing its fall in the first place.

Hot olive oil was thought to work; thereby suggesting Italy, we presume, as the birthplace of the original 'greasy kid's stuff'.

Vinegar was thought to work and cortizone and watercress. Sulphur and acid compounds have been tested, as well as opium and essence of roses blended into an ointment of wine and oil of acacia.

Indeed, for every 'specialist' who sings the praises of organic vegetable juices another is waiting in the wings to tell you about the hair-raising success of magic massage, ultraviolet rays, high-frequency waves, special diet, or – wonder of wonders – a special, electric heating cap.

But search no more!

If you are bald or balding, the United States Government offers the following advice:

'Forget it!'

Baldness in men is an inherited trait, and no product can make hair grow back on a bald head or keep the remaining strands from falling, says the Food and Drug Administration.

The administration, which regularly reviews the claims and effectiveness of non-prescription drugs, has in fact proposed a ban from the market of all hair-restoration products and potions. The prohibition would take effect after a ninety-day period for public comments on the move.

An advisory panel of doctors reporting to the administration delivered its verdict loud and clear.

'Nothing,' they said, 'done to the hair shaft once it emerges from the surface of the scalp will influence hair growth.'

And that's that!

Maybe. . .

9

What the Hecht! or the Second Best Bald Joke in the World

American writer Ben Hecht, in *A Child of the Century*, tells the poignant story of actor Julius Tannen and his search for work. Tannen, pounding the pavement and knocking on doors to the point of giving up, is finally offered a chance to read for the part of a tough, big-city newspaper editor. The reading is arranged by friends who care. Donning his very best suit, shining his very best shoes and wearing his very best tie, Tannen stops in the hallway of his home to measure the impact in a mirror there.

He's bald. Totally bald.

And caring very much about the part, he decides to go one step further and pulls from his wardrobe a headful of hair in the form of a very expensive toupee.

He arrives on time. The producer, after the necessary preliminary conversation, asks him to read.

And he reads, and reads, with all the passion and feeling he can muster.

The producer listens, as carefully as a producer should. And when Tannen has finished reading the rôle, the producer – despite all of his promises to Tannen's friends – says simply, 'I'm sorry, Mr Tannen, my problem is that I've always visualized the editor of this newspaper as a bald-headed man.'

Julius is ecstatic. 'Well, sir,' he responds, while slowly removing the wig, 'I think I can satisfy you.'

The producer sits, studies Tannen's polished skull; then shakes his head and mutters:

'I'm sorry, Mr Tannen ... I simply cannot picture you as a bald-headed man.'

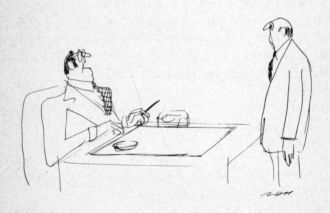

"*Nothing personal, Carstairs. We're firing all bald personnel.*"

10
Test Your Virility

Recent findings suggesting that the bald and balding are simply further along the evolutionary scale than apes or other hairy primates are bound to cause controversy. So too are startling

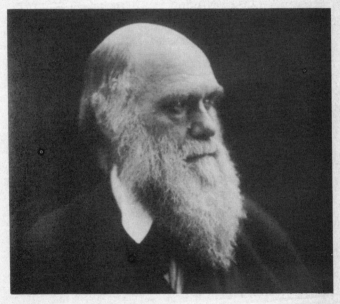

statistics emerging from various hair-and-penis-thickness studies being conducted at private clinics around the world.

The debate will continue.

Why do eunuchs have full heads of hair?

Why do the bald and balding 'perform' so well?

Why do science-fiction writers seem convinced that the truly intelligent aliens, who will inevitably visit us from other worlds, will be without hair? (Yoda, the folk aboard the spaceship in *Close Encounters*, E.T. . . .)

Papers will be published.

Books will be written.

Scientists, sexologists and theorists of every stripe will ruminate, speculate and pontificate in print, in person, on radio and on TV.

But alas, for the layman, the scientific community will undoubtedly manage, once again, to report its findings without once commenting on the one aspect of this overall debate which most concerns us all: *virility*.

Fortunately, our worries and questions about virility can be easily answered and put to rest (with the obvious advantages of confidentiality, and in the privacy of our own homes) by means of the following questionnaire.

So, in the language of the day, go rate yourself.

Taylor's Virility Guide and Questionnaire

1. Do you own a hair brush?

   ☐ yes *(Score 5)*
   ☐ no *(Score 10)*

2. Do you own a comb?

   ☐ yes *(Score 5)*
   ☐ no *(Score 10)*

3. Do you own a hair drier?

   ☐ yes *(Score 5)*
   ☐ no *(Score 15)*

4. How often do you brush or comb your hair?

   ☐ once a day *(Score 15)*
   ☐ twice a day *(Score 10)*
   ☐ more than three times daily *(Score 5)*
   ☐ never *(Score 20)*

5. How often do you get a haircut?

   ☐ once a day *(Score 5)*
   ☐ once a week *(Score 10)*
   ☐ once a month *(Score 15)*
   ☐ once a year *(Score 20)*
   ☐ never *(Score 25)*

6. How many 'hair-care' products do you have in your medicine cabinet?

   ☐ one *(Score 20)*
   ☐ two *(Score 15)*
   ☐ three *(Score 10)*
   ☐ at least a dozen *(Score 5)*
   ☐ none *(Score 25)*

7. Has anyone ever called you 'baldy'?

   ☐ yes *(Score 20)*
   ☐ no *(Score 5)*

8. When did you start losing your hair?

   ☐ a year ago *(Score 10)*
   ☐ two years ago *(Score 15)*
   ☐ more than five years ago *(Score 20)*
   ☐ more than ten years ago *(Score 25)*
   ☐ I was born bald *(Score 30)*
   ☐ yesterday *(Score 5)*

9. Were your parents bald?

   ☐ father *(Score 10)*
   ☐ mother *(Score 15)*
   ☐ both *(Score 25)*

10. How long have you been bald?

   ☐ less than a year *(Score 20)*
   ☐ more than a year *(Score 25)*
   ☐ since birth *(Score 30)*
   ☐ since yesterday *(Score 15)*
   ☐ since this morning *(Score 10)*
   ☐ I have a perfectly good head of hair *(Score 5)*

11. Do women ever tell you that they would like to be bald?

   ☐ yes *(Score 10)*
   ☐ no *(Score 5)*

12. Indicate your head type

☐ hairy as an ape *(Score 5)*
☐ hairy as a fur ball *(Score 10)*
☐ hairy as a peach *(Score 15)*
☐ hairy as an egg *(Score 20)*

Scoring

55–65 – animals of the opposite sex find you interesting and attractive. Game wardens and forest rangers are apt to keep an eye on you when campers and tourists are about. Your dates keep scratching you behind the ears, and throwing sticks for you to fetch.

70–110 – you have a tendency to confuse 'getting a date' with 'cutting one out of the herd'. You dream about Lassie, Flicka, Bambi (if you are very young) and other Hollywood *stars*. Whips and chairs excite you and you just might jump through a ring of fire for a banana.

115–125 – you get your share of dates. You still growl during intercourse, but have finally stopped chasing cars.

130–175 – women have a hard time keeping their hands off you. You have a hard time saying 'no'. Ladies confess strange fantasies. Your phone will ring in about one minute from now.

185–210 – you are sweet, gentle, accommodating, and kind. You are insatiable, untiring and have probably been called 'wonderful' within the past half hour.

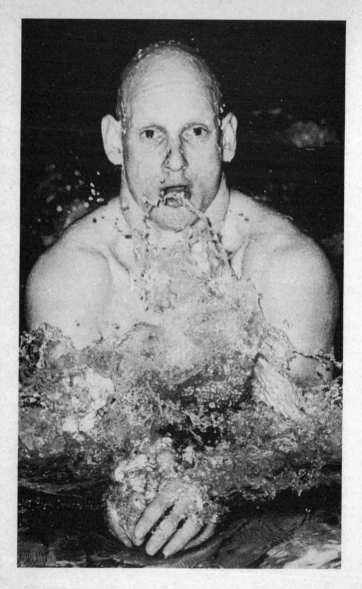

11
Heads I Win!

By now it should come as no surprise to learn that bald sportsmen are in a class of their own – when it comes to staying power, skill and intelligence they're way out ahead. Most of them are also handsome, charming and irresistible . . . .

Pick of the pack in rugby football are Scotland's Jim Cuthbertson and Alistair Biggar. Strong, determined and the baldest players on the pitch they're naturally the men of every match they play in.

To motor-racing fans everywhere Niki Lauda is the undisputed champion of the racetrack, while in Britain Stirling Moss is a watchword for speed. When a policeman stops you for speeding and asks, 'Who do you think you are?' you can be sure he isn't thinking of James Hunt.

Darting through the water like a speeding bullet, Olympic swimmer Duncan Goodhew is ideally suited to his element. Smooth, sleek and streamlined, he doesn't give other swimmers a chance . . . .

When it comes to cricket, Geoff Boycott is certainly a name to conjure with. Keeps a cool

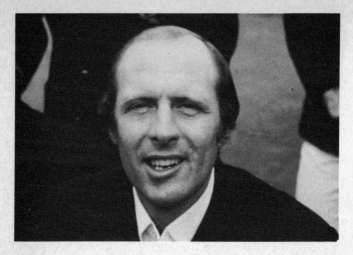

head when others are losing theirs and usually comes up trumps downunder.

Mention English football in any bar around the world and you're still certain to end up talking about one man – Bobby Charlton. A World-Cup player without equal and a footballing legend in his own lifetime. His manager, Sir Matt Busby, was also bald. It's too much to be a coincidence.

Tennis stars come and tennis stars go but none can hold a racket to Bob Hewitt, a world-beating doubles' player. While at Wimbledon, it's good to know that Teddy Tinling's still around to offset some of the more dishevelled mops seen on the Centre Court these days. Dapper, suave and totally bald, he brings elegance and sartorial style to every championship.

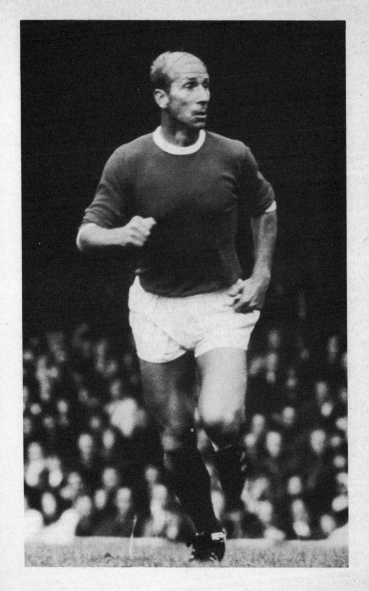

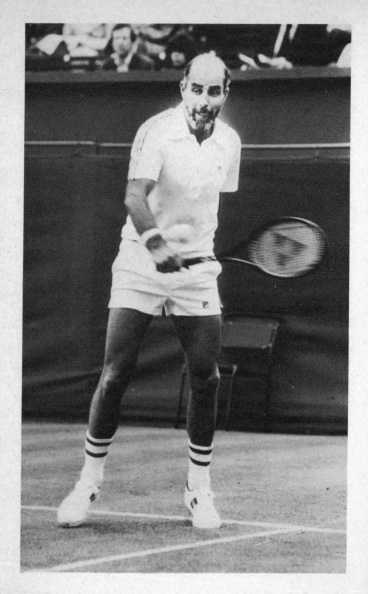

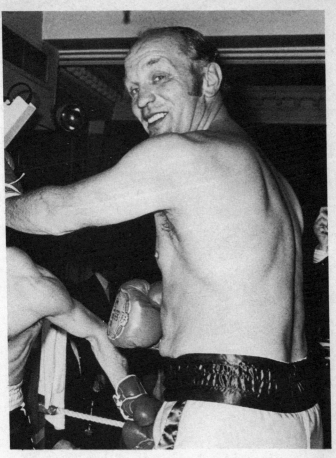

Boxing fans everywhere already *know* that bald is beautiful when it comes to a round in the ring. They've seen Henry Cooper, Marvin Hagler and Earnie Shavers dance and dazzle their way to victory, leaving their rivals out for the count every time!

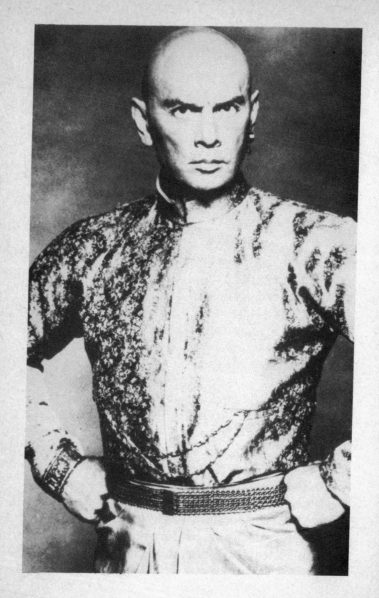

12
Look Ma! No Hair!

Yul Brynner did it in 1951 for *The King and I*. Telly Savalas did it in 1965, when director George Stevens insisted he do it for the rôle of Pontius Pilate in *The Greatest Story Ever Told* – and, as television's lollipop-licking Kojak, has made it his trademark ever since. And while both undoubtedly stand out as the best-known and most popular converts to the world of the bald and beautiful, the shaved head has long been, and remains, a distinguished and glistening part of man's tonsorial repertoire.

It was chic in ancient Egypt for the Pharaohs and even their queens. Dubbed *domus chromus* by the Romans, it was proudly displayed as a mark of power and manliness in the Senate chambers and at the ringside in the Colosseum.

In Elizabethan times, for both sexes, a long intelligent forehead was the fashion of the day, and whether that intelligence was real or not was something only your barber knew for sure.

Jewish orthodoxy once required brides to shave off the hair that adorned their heads as unmarried maidens.

The desire to be bald, it seems, has always been with us – and if the world around us today is any example, the list of those who want to join our ranks will continue to grow for many years to come.

'It's a powerful look, a sexy look,' says Geoffrey Holder, director of the hit musical, *The Wiz*.

Sexy indeed!

New York (where else?), in fact, produced *The Razor's Edge* – a magazine catering to certain gentlemen whose glasses fog at the sight of ladies minus locks.

Indian actress Persis Khambatla did it to play Ilia in the movie *Star Trek*.

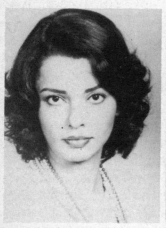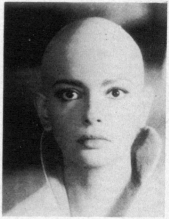

Stratford Johns did it as *Annie's* Daddy Warbucks (on the stage), as did Albert Finney (for the film).

Skinheads did it, causing a boom in barber shops everywhere.

While punks do it (totally, or in the classic Mohican style) depending on the fad or fancy of the day.

Whatever the reasons – sexiness, a look of power or intelligence, a mark of distinction or rebelliousness – everybody, it seems, wants to get in on our act.

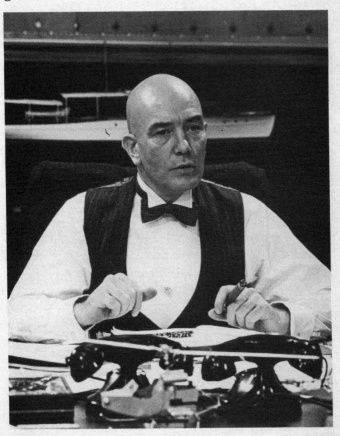

> **Freedom's just another word**
> **for nothin' left to lose.**
> KRIS KRISTOFFERSON

13
The Top Ten Tops

In a world so filled with beautiful people, the task of picking the Top Ten Tops – of placing one person ahead of another, as it were – isn't an easy one. There are files to be combed, and you must brush up on just *who's who*.

And while our choices are, ultimately, subjective, our basic guideline in selecting the hairlines that follow was that the candidates should be part of the contemporary world – thereby eliminating many great pates from the past – and that they should be 'natural', thereby eliminating those who have shaved or sheared their way into our flock. (See Chapter 12.)

Finally, our decision-making process demanded, above all else, that the gentlemen who shine from the following pages bring dignity and style to our ranks – that they spread pride and joy while shedding hair so that generations to come will know that BALD IS BEAUTIFUL indeed.

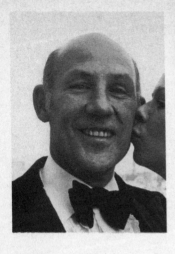 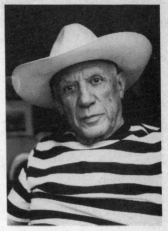

1 *Stirling Moss*
A natural choice for pole position. Cool as a cucumber, as handsome as a bald man should be, and without doubt, the fastest bald head in the world.

2 *Pablo Picasso*
You ever hear of him before he went bald? Of course not! To Pablo then, a sexy second spot in this Ten Tops hit-parade for making the world a more beautiful place.

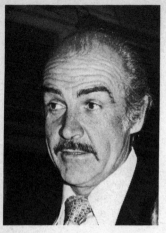

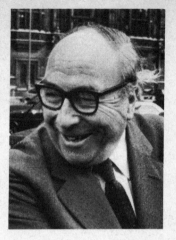

3 *Sean Connery*
For 007, gracefully
ageing right along
with the rest of us;
and for removing his
hairpiece in *Never Say
Never Again*.

4 *Roy Jenkins*
People have been
talking about a new
party in Britain since
Wedgwood Benn was
in short trousers, but
it took a bald
politician to make it
all possible!

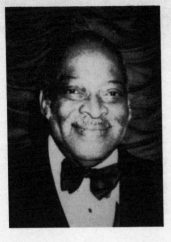

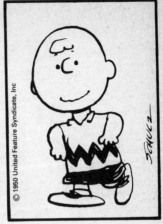

© 1950 United Feature Syndicate, Inc

5 *Count Basie*
For *April In Paris, One O' Clock Jump* and all the carefree, hairfree jazz of our lives.

6 *Charlie Brown*
No superstar on the football pitch, but *good grief*, doesn't he give his all? Chuck's top with us for the simple reason that he has never once complained, he's there to cheer you up when you're feeling down and is the ultimate proof that premature balding needn't age you a single day.

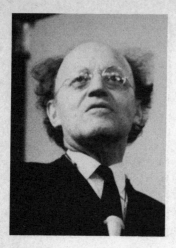 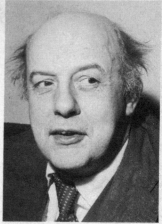

7 *Lord Longford*
A tireless campaigner
and peerless Peer.
Living proof that
baldness is next to
Godliness.

8 *Sir John Betjeman*
The only Poet
Laureate people have
read for pleasure
since Lord Tennyson.
Follows in a long line
of bald bards from
Shakespeare to
Wordsworth.

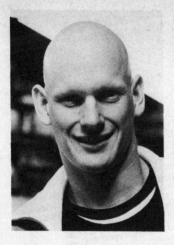

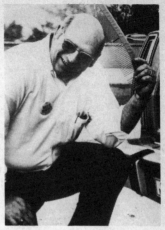

9 *Duncan Goodhew*
Young, gifted and
bald – what a
combination!

10 *John T. Capps III*
The founder and
president of the
BHMA (Bald-Headed
Men of America) – a
club dedicated to the
simple philosophy
that 'Bald is
Beautiful', and which
believes that
everyone with less
than a full head of
hair should flaunt it
rather than hide it
under wigs or hair
transplants.

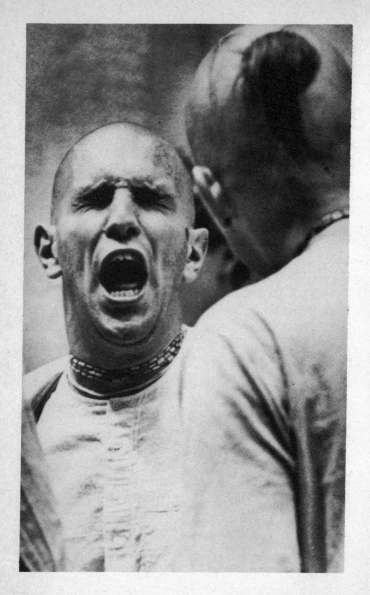

> **A man of my resources cannot presume to have a hair-style – get on and cut it.**
> WINSTON CHURCHILL

14

The Hairy Krishnas and Other Frauds

1 The Mexican Hairless definitely has hair.
2 The electric hairbrush. Despite the suggestion, it's twice as much bother as the old-fashioned kind. A friend of ours purchased one recently, plugged it in and all it did was sit there.
3 Ronald Reagan – nobody's hair is that colour.
4 Yasser Arafat who'd have us believe he wears that kerchief to keep the sand and wind and the rain out of his hair. C'mon Yasser, take it off!
5 The bald-faced lie – a misunderstanding on your part. If it's that easy to spot, the speaker was probably just pulling your leg.
6 Barbers who charge me the same price they'd charge George Harrison.
7 The Hairy Krishnas.

15
A Tall Bald Stranger

Yul Brynner broke the bald barrier as the King of Siam. Telly Savalas did it as the lovable, tough detective Kojak on TV. Warren Mitchell, as Alf Garnett, was television at its very best, proving for all time that baldness grows on movie and television audiences just as easily as hair.

Despite all this, let's not be blinded by the glare of all those movie lights – two television series, and one movie!

Three roles for a group whose number is counted in millions in Britain alone! This is perfect nonsense and the sort of thing the bald and balding have had to live with since the days of silent films.

Show us a romantic lead that couldn't be played by any one of us.

Show us a leading lady who wouldn't jump at a chance to be a gleam in the eye of a man who can really take a shine to her.

And the film industry isn't alone – when was the last time you read a novel with a dashing, virile hero who was bald?

Are Mills and Boon and other publishers *that*

unaware of the fantasies of the suburban
housewife?

And what about the horoscopes – why must
the stranger always be tall and dark?

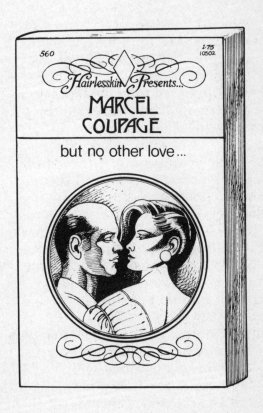

16
The Samson Myth

We've heard for years of Samson's strength,
His height, and weight, his hair's great length;
But nowhere does the Book explain
That Samson didn't have much brain.
How else, pray tell to understand
Why this strong man who ruled the land
By massacring Philistines
And setting fires, and killing lions,
Would take a vow of don't's and do's
Forbidding haircuts, girls, and booze?
It helps us know and comprehend
Delilah's quandary to the end.
She poured him drink and cut his hair
And helped remove his underwear.
She taught him things he didn't know
But three vows down and none to go
Is field position none too fine
When playing with the Philistine.
His strength now gone from all that play
They simply carted him away.
They told him not to move at all.
They bound him to the Temple wall,
The very Temple where they dwelled.
(His hair grew back, his muscles swelled.)
Escaping didn't cross his mind

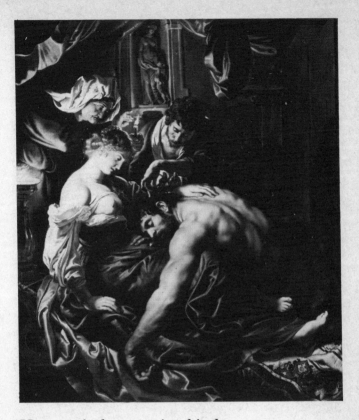

He wasn't the escaping kind.
He didn't try to free his wrists,
Or wriggle free with clever twists.
Instead he used his brain, and QED,
He brought the house down on his head.
Now Samson and his hair are gone,
His three-fold vow and all his brawn.
Delilah lives on anyhow,
She's Patron Saint of Barbers now.

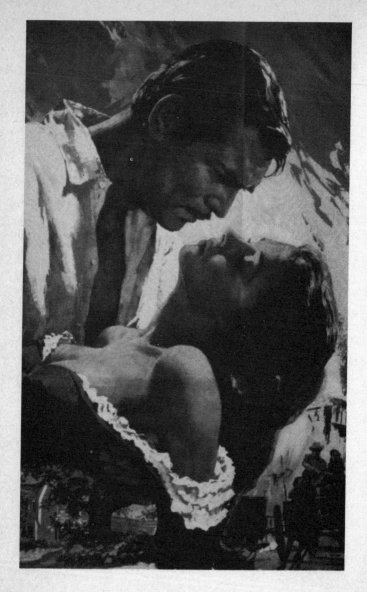

17

Frankly Scarlett, I'd Rather Be Bald

Did you know? That the human scalp produces an average of 0.35 millimetres – a bit more than one hundredth of an inch – of hair per day, and that the energy required of the body's metabolism to produce this amount of hair is greater than that required to produce any other bodily tissues. (No wonder those guys look so tired most of the time.)

Did you know? That the Lamont method of hair replacement developed in 1957 involves cutting out your sideburns and using them as flaps of skin and hair to sew across your former hairline.

Did you know? That Doctors Iturrospe and Arufe of Buenos Aires are the inventors of another system which involves, like face lifting, the surgical removal of a strip from the middle of your bald spot; the side fringes are then pulled closer together.

A bald-headed man is very exciting
AIDA GREY

18
Off the Top of My Head

From 'Thoughts on the Top of My Head: the facts. The bare facts. The bald truth' By Guy Martin, *Esquire*

'Since balding in real life is infinitely more difficult than balding on paper, I include a few points of balding etiquette; suggestions, really, to help you get over some of the rough spots.

- You bald because you inherited an overload of testosterone. Use it.
- Learn balding history so that you may speak with authority at cocktails. Marcel Duchamp, Henry Miller, Henry Adams, Haile Selassie are balding history. Philip Roth and Terry Bradshaw don't deserve it. Menachem Begin doesn't either.
- Appear in a tuxedo as often as possible.
- Take a vacation in Japan to coincide with the annual Bright Head Contest, the beauty pageant for bald men.
- Have one round, shiny, expensive object in a prominent place in your house.
- Bring a baby to your next social engagement.'

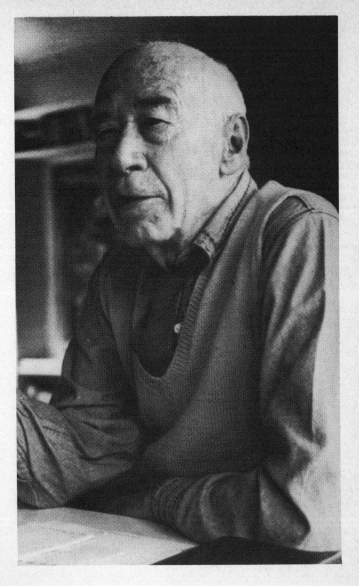

Bald is Beautiful

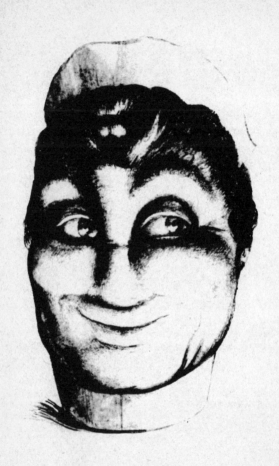

86

19
Taking it on the Chin

Is it possible that the increasing number of beards on city streets and in offices throughout the world is a desperate try at one more style of cover-up?

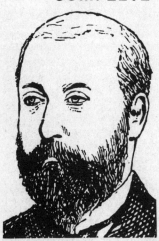

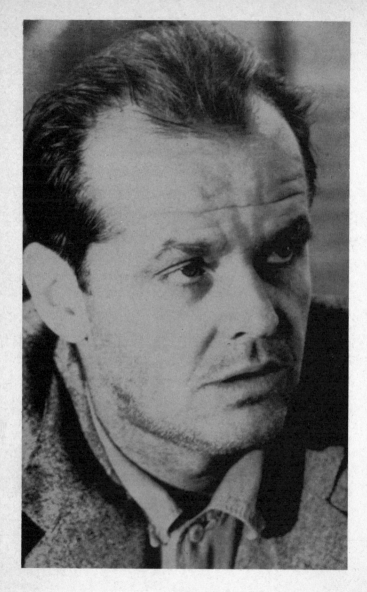